Table of Contents

INTRODUCTION 5
CHAPTER ONE 8
What is CBD? 8
Health Benefits of CBD 12
Medical uses 15
Pharmacology 17
    Pharmacodynamics 17
    Pharmacokinetics 18
    Pharmaceutical preparations 18
    Chemistry 19
    Biosynthesis 20
    Food and beverage 20
    Plant sources 22
    Non-psychoactivity 23
Legal status 24
    United Nations 24
    Australia 25
    Canada 25
    European Union 26
    Sweden 27

New Zealand 27

United Kingdom 28

United States 29

Switzerland 33

Research 34

The Fundamentals of Cannabidiol 34

Cannabidiol is Not Psychoactive 34

Cannabidiol is Legal Almost Everywhere 35

Cannabidiol Can Come From Hemp or Marijuana Plants . 37

Breeders Are Crafting Specialized CBD-Dominant Weed Strains 39

What Does Cannabidiol Actually Do? 40

How Does Cannabidiol Interact With The Body? 41

What CBD Can Really Do—And The Research Backing It Up 43

CBD Can Stop Epileptic Seizures 43

CBD Can Treat Serious Neurological Diseases Like Alzheimer's, Multiple Sclerosis, and Parkinson's 44

CBD Can Relieve Pain 45

CBD Can Fight Cancer 46

CBD Can Reduce Inflammation 47

CBD Can Treat Mood Disorders 48

What Can CBD Do For Recreational Users? 48

- CBD Can Produce A Smoother, More Balanced High 49
- The Most Popular CBD Products Available Today 51
- The Future Of Cannabidiol: The Future Of Healing? 52
- CHAPTER TWO 54
- How much CBD is in a gummy? 54
  - Take time to get your dose right 54
  - How to find the best CBD gummies 56
  - CBD Gummies—What's Real and What's Fake 58
- FAQs about CBD gummies 60
  - Is CBD safe? 60
  - Are CBD gummies legal in the United States? 60
  - How many CBD gummies should I eat? 61
  - Will I fail a drug test if I eat CBD gummies? 62
  - Where can I buy CBD gummies? 63
  - The Differences Between CBD Gummies and CBD Oil 63
  - CBD Gummies Are The Same As CBD Oil! 64
  - CBD Gummies Are Different From CBD Oil 67
  - Increasing Popularity of CBD Gummies 68
  - How to pick the right CBD gummies 72
  - Note 75
- Our Review Methodology 77
  - Is the CBD gummy full-spectrum or an isolate? 78

Does this brand operate in a state where marijuana is legal? 78

Do I want a brand that does one thing great or has everything I need? 79

Does this brand have assistance programs and military discounts available? 80

CHAPTER THREE 81

CBD Gummies for Anxiety 81

CBD Anxiety & Depression Studies 81

Using CBD Gummies For Anxiety & Depression 83

Why Do People Choose CBD Gummies Over Other Forms Of CBD? 85

CHAPTER FOUR 94

CONCLUSION 94

INTRODUCTION

CBD and CBD Oil has become some of the most sought-after medicines on the market today. Not only is it able to treat a wide range of ailments ranging from cancer to arthritis, CBD is known to be effective without causing any obvious side effects. It can be used safely in the long-term without causing addiction and dependence.

There are tons of ways to use CBD, and one of the most popular is to use CBD gummies. These products provide patients with a tasty and fun way to medicate themselves. CBD is attractive to a number of people because it presents a holistic alternative to a lot of pharmaceutical medications. Many people find that their pharmaceuticals may be effective for treating a problem on the surface, but the side effects often compete with the benefits and in the long-run the illness is rarely treated. CBD gummies, on the other hand, can help people manage the symptoms of their illnesses without actually becoming dependent on a drug or overwhelmed by side effects. This provides a unique opportunity to actually heal the root of the problem.

One of the most popular uses for CBD gummies and other forms of CBD is for helping people manage anxiety. Many people were baffled by the implications of this, particularly because THC is well-known for causing anxiety in many people. Folks were wondering how a cannabinoid – especially one so similar to THC – could be used for fighting anxiety.

CBD has been shown to be useful for fighting all sorts of anxiety, ranging from generalized anxiety to panic disorder. Many have found success using a vape pen to help them manage acute panic attacks. CBD has even been shown to help fight anxiety associated with serious conditions like post-traumatic stress disorder.

CHAPTER ONE

What is CBD?

An acronym for cannabidiol, it's a type of cannabinoid found in the cannabis. There are over 400 chemical compounds present in the hemp. Out of those 400, around 60 chemicals are totally unique to cannabis including hemp. Cannabidiol is one of those compounds that doctors frequently use for therapeutic intervention. The great thing about CBD is that it carries no psychoactive propertiesunlike THC (tetrahydrocannabinol). That is why you don't get to experience the 'high' associated with THC based products. In fact, CBD counters the effect of THC and helps with withdrawal symptoms. It's also supposed to help with chronic pains, inflammation, headaches, and myriad other health problems. This is the reason CBD is not banned in most places. Patients consume

CBD in a variety of forms like oil, tincture, vapes, wax concentrates, powder, capsule, etc. And, now they can avail its health benefits by consuming it in the form of candy.

Marijuana contains high levels of THC, a psychoactive chemical that's responsible for making you feel "high." CBD sold legally in the United States has less than .03 percent THC, which isn't enough THC to make a rodent high. It's safe for consumption for all ages, and clinical and anecdotal research shows its many health benefits. In fact, the FDA recently approved a CBD-based drug called Epidolex, which is a drug used by children and adults to reduce the frequency and severity of seizures.

CBD is available in many different forms. It can be applied topically through oils and lotions, but it's more common to take it orally through gummies, beverages, or capsules. GBD gummies are probably the most popular because they're convenient and tasty. The sweet, fruity flavors of these gummies remove the earthy taste that many people don't like, making it easier and more enjoyable to eat.

CBD and Your Endocannabinoid System

In a moment, you'll read all about the many health benefits of CBD, but it's useful to first examine how CBD works within your body and to avoid misconceptions. It does not in any way alter your cognitive state, so you don't have to worry about being "out of it" or "high" when you'd rather have your wits about you.

Instead, it works in tandem with your body's endocannabinoid system. This system is responsible for receiving transmissions from the cannabinoids within your body. These signals express sensations like pain and contribute to causing inflammation in the body.

CBD blocks some of the receptors in this system, preventing pain signals from reaching the brain. It works very similarly to non-steroid-anti-inflammatory drugs (NSAID) like ibuprofen, dulling the pain and negative symptoms associated with injuries or stress.

When using CBD gummies, it's important to choose products in which CBD is the main ingredient. The gummies you buy online should be low in THC to eliminate psychoactive properties. Some gummies have more sugar and flavoring in them than they do CBD, which dulls the effectiveness of the drug. When taken in the right dose, CBD typically works quickly and has long-lasting effects.

Health Benefits of CBD

The clinical studies on CBD are minimal, thanks to the controversy surrounding them. Much of the research has been performed on rodents. However, research clinics are becoming more familiar with CBD's potential benefits and are seeking funding to perform human trials to prove the effectiveness in the drug.

Rodent studies as well as countless stories and human experiences have shown extremely positive effects of taking CBD for health and wellness. Some of the most common benefits include:

• Relieved Pain

• Lessened Inflammation

• Cancer Prevention and Delay

• Prevention of Serious Illnesses and Diseases

- Reduced Mental Health Problems

- Relieved Stress

- Better Sleep

Some of the most compelling research points to CBD's ability to minimize anxiety. Those who have suffered from anxiety for their entire lives with little respite report amazing results from using CBD gummies. They report feeling almost instantly calm, and they rave about the convenience of taking gummies at any time without hassle.

CBD is becoming more accepted in the healthcare community thanks to studies that have proven CBD to be an effective supplement for reducing the frequency and severity of seizures for epilepsy patients. The FDA recently approved the first CBD-based drug called Epidolex that's used to treat this disorder with minimal side effects.

Because it has proven so effective in this situation and the side effects are so minimal, many pharmaceutical companies have begun taking interest in CBD as an effective drug. Studies are currently being performed to prove the effectiveness of the supplement when used to treat many of the conditions listed above. It won't be long before the world is well-versed in the empirical benefits of taking CBD.

Medical uses

Epilepsy

There has been little high-quality research into the use of cannabidiol for epilepsy. The limited available evidence primarily focuses on refractory epilepsy in children. While the results of using medical-grade cannabidiol in combination with conventional medication shows some promise, they did not lead to seizures being eliminated, and were associated with some minor adverse effects.

Other uses

Preliminary research on other possible therapeutic uses for cannabidiol include several neurological disorders, but the findings have not been confirmed by sufficient high-quality clinical research to establish such uses in clinical practice.

Side effects

Preliminary research indicates that cannabidiol may reduce adverse effects of THC, particularly those causing intoxication and sedation, but only at high doses. Safety studies of cannabidiol showed it is well-tolerated, but may cause tiredness, diarrhea, or changes in appetite as common adverse effects. Epidiolex documentation lists sleepiness, insomnia and poor quality sleep, decreased appetite, diarrhea, and fatigue.

Potential interactions

Laboratory evidence indicated that cannabidiol may reduce THC clearance, increasing plasma concentrations which may raise THC availability to receptors and enhance its effect in a dose-dependent manner. In vitro, cannabidiol inhibited receptors affecting the activity of voltage-dependent sodium and potassium channels, which may affect neural activity. A small clinical trialreported that CBD partially inhibited the CYP2C-catalyzed hydroxylation of THC to 11-OH-THC. Little is known about potential drug interactions, but CBD-mediates a decrease in clobazam metabolism.

Pharmacology

Pharmacodynamics

Cannabidiol has low affinity for the cannabinoid CB1 and CB2 receptors, although it can act as an antagonist of CB1/CB2 agonists despite this low affinity. Cannabidiol may be an antagonist of GPR55, a G protein-coupled receptor and putative cannabinoid receptor that is expressed in the caudate nucleus and putamen in the brain. It also may act as an inverse agonist of GPR3, GPR6, and GPR12. CBD has been shown to act as a serotonin 5-HT1A receptor partial agonist. It is an allosteric modulator of the μ- and δ-opioid receptors as well. The pharmacological effects of CBD may involve PPARγ agonism and intracellular calcium release.

Pharmacokinetics

The oral bioavailability of CBD is 13 to 19%, while its bioavailability via inhalation is 11 to 45% (mean 31%).The elimination half-life of CBD is 18–32 hours. Cannabidiol is metabolized in the liver as well as in the intestines by CYP2C19 and CYP3A4 enzymes, and UGT1A7, UGT1A9, and UGT2B7 isoforms. CBD may have a wide margin in dosing.

Pharmaceutical preparations

Nabiximols (brand name Sativex) is a patented medicine containing CBD and THC in equal proportions. The drug was approved by Health Canada in 2005 for prescription to treat central neuropathic pain in multiple sclerosis, and in 2007 for cancer related pain. In New Zealand, Sativex is "approved for use as an add-on treatment for symptom improvement in people with moderate to severe spasticity due to multiple sclerosis who have not responded adequately to other anti-spasticity medication."

Epidiolex is an orally administered cannabidiol solution. It was approved in 2018 by the US Food and Drug Administration for treatment of two rare forms of childhood epilepsy, Lennox-Gastaut syndrome and Dravet syndrome.

Chemistry

Cannabidiol is insoluble in water but soluble in organic solvents such as pentane. At room temperature, it is a colorless crystalline solid. In strongly basic media and the presence of air, it is oxidized to a quinone. Under acidic conditions it cyclizes to THC, which also occurs during pyrolysis (smoking). The synthesis of cannabidiol has been accomplished by several research groups.

Biosynthesis

Cannabis produces CBD-carboxylic acid through the same metabolic pathway as THC, until the next to last step, where CBDA synthase performs catalysis instead of THCA synthase.

Food and beverage

Food and beverage products containing CBD were introduced in the United States in 2017.[Hemp seed ingredients which do not naturally contain THC or CBD (but which may be contaminated with trace amounts on the outside during harvesting) were declared by the FDA as GRAS in December

2018. CBD itself has not been declared GRAS, and under U.S. federal law is illegal to sell as a food, dietary supplement, or animal feed. State laws vary considerably as non-medical cannabis and derived products have been legalized in some jurisdictions in the 2010s.

Similar to energy drinks and protein bars which may contain vitamin or herbal additives, food and beverage items can be infused with CBD as an alternative means of ingesting the substance. In the United States, numerous products are marketed as containing CBD, but in reality contain little or none. Some companies marketing CBD-infused food products with claims that are similar to the effects of prescription drugs have received warning letters from the Food and Drug Administration for making unsubstantiated health claims. In February 2019, the New York City Department of Health announced plans to fine restaurants that sell food or drinks containing CBD, beginning in October 2019.

Plant sources

Selective breeding of cannabis plants has expanded and diversified as commercial and therapeutic markets develop. Some growers in the US succeeded in lowering the proportion of CBD-to-THC to accommodate customers who preferred varietals that were more mind-altering due to the higher THC and lower CBD content. In the US, hemp is classified by the federal government as cannabis containing no more than 0.3% THC by dry weight. This classification was established in the 2018 Farm Bill and was refined to include hemp-sourced extracts, cannabinoids, and derivatives in the definition of hemp.

Non-psychoactivity

CBD does not appear to have any psychotropic ("high") effects such as those caused by Δ9-THC in marijuana, but may[specify] have anti-anxiety and anti-psychotic effects. As the legal landscape and understanding about the differences in medical cannabinoids unfolds, experts are working to distinguish "medical marijuana" (with varying degrees of psychotropic effects and deficits in executive function) – from "medical CBD therapies" which would commonly present as having a reduced or non-psychoactive side-effect profile.

Various strains of "medical marijuana" are found to have a significant variation in the ratios of CBD-to-THC, and are known to contain other non-psychotropic cannabinoids. Any psychoactive marijuana, regardless of its CBD content, is derived from the flower (or bud) of the genus Cannabis. As defined by U.S. federal law, non-psychoactive hemp (also commonly-termed industrial hemp), regardless of its CBD content, is any part of the cannabis plant, whether growing or not, containing a Δ-9 tetrahydrocannabinol concentration of no more than 0.3% on a dry-weight basis. Certain standards are required for legal growing, cultivating, and producing the hemp plant. The Colorado Industrial Hemp Program registers growers of industrial hemp and samples crops to verify that the dry-weight THC concentration does not exceed 0.3%.

Legal status

United Nations

Cannabidiol is not scheduled under the Convention on Psychotropic Substances or any other UN drug treaty. In 2018, the World Health Organization recommended that CBD remain unscheduled.

Australia

Prescription medicine (Schedule 4) for therapeutic use containing 2 per cent (2.0%) or less of other cannabinoids commonly found in cannabis (such as Δ9-THC). A schedule 4 drug under the SUSMP is Prescription Only Medicine, or Prescription Animal Remedy – Substances, the use or supply of which should be by or on the order of persons permitted by State or Territory legislation to prescribe and should be available from a pharmacist on prescription.

Following a change in legislation in 2017, CBD was changed from a schedule 9 drug to a schedule 4 drug, meaning that it is legally available in Australia.

Canada

In October 2018, cannabidiol became legal for recreational and medical use.

European Union

In 2019, the European Commission announced that CBD and other cannabinoids would be classified as "novel foods", meaning that CBD products would require authorization under the EU Novel Food Regulation stating: because "this product was not used as a food or food ingredient before 15 May 1997, before it may be placed on the market in the EU as a food or food ingredient, a safety assessment under the Novel Food Regulation is required." The recommendation – applying to CBD extracts, synthesized CBD, and all CBD products, including CBD oil – was scheduled for a final ruling by the European Commission in March 2019. If approved, manufacturers of CBD products would be required to conduct safety tests and prove safe consumption, indicating that CBD products would not be eligible for legal commerce until at least 2021.

Cannabidiol is listed in the EU Cosmetics Ingredient Database (CosIng). However, the listing of an ingredient, assigned with an INCI name, in CosIng does not mean it is to be used in cosmetic products or is approved for such use.

Several industrial hemp varieties can be legally cultivated in Western Europe. A variety such as "Fedora 17" has a cannabinoid profile consistently around 1%, with THC less than 0.3%.

Sweden
CBD is classified as a medical product in Sweden.

New Zealand
In 2017 the government made changes to the regulations so that restrictions would be removed, which meant a doctor was able to prescribe cannabidiol to patients.

The passing of the Misuse of Drugs (Medicinal Cannabis) Amendment Act in December 2018 means cannabidiol is no longer a controlled drug in New Zealand, but is a prescription medicine under the Medicines Act provided the product contains no more than two percent THC of total CBD.

United Kingdom

Cannabidiol, in an oral-mucosal spray formulation combined with delta-9-tetrahydrocannabinol, is a product available (by prescription only until 2017) for relief of severe spasticity due to multiple sclerosis (where other anti-spasmodicshave not been effective).

Until 2017, products containing cannabidiol marketed for medical purposes were classed as medicines by the UK regulatory body, the Medicines and Healthcare products Regulatory

Agency (MHRA) and could not be marketed without regulatory approval for the medical claims. As of 2018, cannabis oil is legal to possess, buy, and sell in the UK, providing the product does not contain more than 0.3% THC and is not advertised as providing a medicinal benefit.

In January 2019, the UK Food Standards Agency indicated it would regard CBD products, including CBD oil, as a novel food in the UK, having no history of use before May 1997, and indicating such products must have authorization and proven safety before being marketed.

United States

As of April 2019, CBD extracted from marijuana remains a Schedule I Controlled Substance, and is not approved as a prescription drug, dietary supplement, or allowed for interstate commerce in the United States. CBD derived from hemp (with

0.3% THC or lower) was delisted as a federally scheduled substance by the 2018 Farm Bill. FDA regulations still apply: hemp CBD is legal to sell as a cosmetics ingredient, but despite a common misconception, because it is an active ingredient in an FDA-approved drug, cannot be sold under federal law as an ingredient in food, dietary supplements, or animal food. It is a common misconception that the legal ability to sell hemp (which may contain CBD) makes CBD legal.

In September 2018, following its approval by the FDA for rare types of childhood epilepsy, Epidiolex was rescheduled (by the Drug Enforcement Administration) as a Schedule V drug to allow for its prescription use. This allows GW Pharmaceuticals to sell Epidiolex, but it does not apply broadly and all other CBD-containing products remain Schedule

I drugs. Epidiolex still requires rescheduling in some states before it can be prescribed in those states.

In 2013 a CNN program that featured Charlotte's Web cannabis brought increased attention to the use of CBD in the treatment of seizure disorders. Since then, 16 states have passed laws to allow the use of CBD products with a doctor's recommendation (instead of a prescription) for treatment of certain medical conditions. This is in addition to the 30 states that have passed comprehensive medical cannabis laws, which allow for the use of cannabis products with no restrictions on THC content. Of these 30 states, eight have legalized the use and sale of cannabis products without requirement for a doctor's recommendation.

Some manufacturers ship CBD products nationally, an illegal action which the FDA did not enforce in

2018, with CBD remaining the subject of an FDA investigational new drug evaluation, and is not considered legal as a dietary supplement or food ingredient as of December 2018. Federal illegality has made it difficult historically to conduct research on CBD. CBD is openly sold in head shops and health food stores in some states where such sales have not been explicitly legalized.

The 2014 Farm Bill[82] legalized the sale of "non-viable hemp material" grown within states participating in the Hemp Pilot Program. This legislation defined hemp as cannabis containing less than 0.3% of THC delta-9, grown within the regulatory framework of the Hemp Pilot Program. The 2018 Farm Bill allowed for interstate commerce of hemp derived products, though these products still fall under the purview of the FDA.

Switzerland

While THC remains illegal, CBD is not subject to the Swiss Narcotic Acts because this substance does not produce a comparable psychoactive effect. Cannabis products containing less than 1% THC can be sold and purchased legally.

Research

As of 2016, there was only limited high-quality evidence for cannabidiol having any neurological effect in people.

The Fundamentals of Cannabidiol

Perhaps the only thing more complex than the biochemistry of cannabis is its pharmacology. The ways weed interacts with the human body are exceedingly intricate. And the truth is we don't know as much as we should about those interactions—at least not yet.

Nevertheless, we do know some of the basics. So here's your fundamental fact sheet about Cannabidiol.

Cannabidiol is Not Psychoactive

One of the most crucially important qualities of CBD is its lack of psycho-activity. In layperson's terms, this means that cannabidiol won't get you high. Unlike THC, the cannabinoid with the legendary power of producing euphoric sensations, Cannabidiol is inert.

So when taken on its own, users experience none of the sensations of being stoned. And this is the single most important property of the cannabinoid from the medical—and legal—perspective.

Cannabidiol is Legal Almost Everywhere

Because CBD doesn't get you high, products that contain only this cannabinoid can skirt the legal ban on marijuana.

Technically speaking, its THC—the cannabinoid that gets you high—which is illicit. When you take a drug test, the aim is to detect THC in your body, not "cannabis." If you possessed weed without any THC in it, technically you wouldn't be in violation of the law. Because "weed" without THC has a different name: hemp. And the rules governing hemp are quite different from the restrictions placed on cannabis.

In fact, every state that has yet to legalize marijuana for medical use has some kind of law allowing people to obtain and use CBD-only (or low-THC) products for medical or therapeutic purposes. And in most cases, that means obtaining Cannabidiol from hemp, rather than cannabis flowers.

In places with legal medical marijuana programs, CBD products are widely available and easy to find.

Cannabidiol Can Come From Hemp or Marijuana Plants

There are two main sources of CBD: hemp plants and marijuana. Where a given product comes from depends on the legal status of marijuana in a particular state.

If medical marijuana is illegal in a given state, THC levels determine whether a CBD product is illicit or not. In most places, the limit is extremely low. We're talking under 1 percent THC, with some states opting for a cap as low as 0.3 percent. In this case, the only source that would work is hemp, and CBD products will, therefore, be hemp-derived.

In other places, limits can be higher. Delaware, for example, allows CBD oil to contain up to 5 percent THC. But that's still not enough to get anyone very high.

Sourcing and legality questions aside, the general consensus has it that CBD derived from marijuana is both more potent and more effective.

Many attribute this phenomenon to the "entourage effect," or the theory that one cannabinoid can do its job better when it works together with its companion cannabinoids. Extracting Cannabidiol from cannabis flowers helps keep these other cannabinoids intact, which is why people prefer it over hemp-derived products.

In other words, the source matters. And the buds of the cannabis plant have a richer and wider complement of cannabinoids compared to hemp leaves. So while we're on the topic, here's a quick rundown of the best CBD-only and CBD-dominant strains of cannabis out there.

Breeders Are Crafting Specialized CBD-Dominant Weed Strains

The demand for medical-grade cannabidiol has spurred breeders and growers to pursue new strain genetics that promote cannabidiol production. These strains don't attempt to eliminate THC. Instead, they increase the ratio of CBD to THC, allowing the effects of cannabidiol to shine through.

- Katelyn Faith: named after the 8-year-old for whom it was created, Katelyn Faith boasts a 34-to-1 cannabidiol to THC ratio, making it one of the most CBD-rich strains in the world.

- Harlequin: A legendary medical strain which weighs in at a 5:2 ratio.

- ACDC: This widely available strain consistently tops 19 percent cannabidiol.

- Remedy: As the name suggests, a potent healing strain with an impressive 15:1 cannabidiol ratio.

- Cannatonic: At a perfect 1:1 ratio of CBD to THC, this strain achieves an optimal ensemble effect for medical patients also seeking the benefits of THC.

- Charlotte's Web: Interestingly, this "strain" isn't marijuana at all. Rather, it's a proprietary hemp plant that produces buds with just the cannabidiol cannabinoid.

What Does Cannabidiol Actually Do?

We've covered the details of what cannabidiol is, its basic properties, and where it comes from. Now, it's time to turn our attention to what this powerful little compound can do.

For good reason, cannabidiol dominates the conversation about the medical applications of cannabis. But that doesn't mean CBD isn't valuable to recreational users. In fact, CBD has some special qualities that can make it an important part of any recreational experience.

How Does Cannabidiol Interact With The Body?

All of the 60-plus cannabinoids unique to the plant genus Cannabis interact with our bodies thanks to a network of neurons called the endocannabinoid system.

The endocannabinoid system runs throughout your body. And it's loaded with receptors that bind to the cannabinoids you introduce to your bloodstream when you consume weed.

And it's the chemical interactions of those bonds that create a wide and largely unknown series of responses in your body.

Without distorting the science too much, you could say that human beings are "hard-wired" for weed. The endocannabinoid system runs deep and touches all of the major systems of the body. And that's why weed can do so many things for us, from altering and regulating moods to stimulating appetites and reducing pain.

And even though cannabidiol has no toxicity for humans—meaning, it doesn't make you intoxicated (i.e. high)—it is highly reactive with the endocannabinoid system.

To put things as simply as possible, CBD makes things happen. When it binds to the endocannabinoid system's receptors, it stimulates all kinds of changes in the body.

Most of those changes are incredibly beneficial, and researchers keep uncovering real and potential medical uses for them.

We won't bog you down with the technical minutiae of each of those changes. Instead, here's a quick overview of the major studies and most promising findings about the medical importance of CBD.

What CBD Can Really Do—And The Research Backing It Up

There's no better way to gain an appreciation of just what cannabidiol can do than taking a look at the exciting research behind it. This overview lists the major medical benefits of CBD, then explains the key studies backing them up.

CBD Can Stop Epileptic Seizures

One of the most important CBD studies ever published was a path-breaking study into the efficacy of using CBD as a treatment for epilepsy.

In 2012, researchers with the British Epilepsy Association published a papercalled "Cannabidiol exerts anticonvulsant effects in animal models of the temporal lobe and partial seizures." Their conclusion? "The evidence strongly supports CBD as a therapeutic candidate for a diverse range of human epilepsies."

CBD Can Treat Serious Neurological Diseases Like Alzheimer's, Multiple Sclerosis, and Parkinson's

Researchers are still trying to figure out the exact mechanisms behind neurodegenerative diseases like Alzheimer's. We know it has to do with a protein pathway, and that's exactly the pathway this 2006 study investigates.

Taking a look down to the molecular level, researchers discovered that CBD can actually protect nerve cells from degenerative diseases. Scientists call this CBD's "neuroprotective effect," and it's one of the most promising aspects of the cannabinoid.

CBD Can Relieve Pain

Medical cannabis is quickly becoming the go-to alternative to dangerous and addictive prescription painkillers, like the opioids that are causing an epidemic of overdose deaths in the United States.

A lot of weed's pain-killing power stems from its psychoactive cannabinoid, THC. But cannabidiol is also a potent pain reliever. 2015 saw the most important study to uncover the pain-relieving effects of CBD. In that study, researchers compared cannabidiol to morphine.

To their surprise, CBD worked well in combination with morphine and counteracted the latter's risky side effects. This means cannabidiol can help treat acute pain conditions, along with more long-term benefits.

CBD Can Fight Cancer

It sounds too good to be true. But indeed, pre-clinical trials have shown that cannabidiol has a powerful anti-tumor effect.

The most important study to reveal these powerful tumor-inhibiting effects came out in 2015. In fact, this study looked at a range of non-psychoactive cannabinoids, including, of course, cannabidiol.

In a landmark for medical cannabis research, this study concluded that "CBD slows the progression of many types of cancer, including breast, lung, prostate and colon cancer."

How that works is pretty incredible. Cannabidiol actually makes it harder for cancer cells to grow. In some cases, this causes an increase in cancer cell death. No wonder stories abound about "miracle" CBD cures that shrink tumors.

CBD Can Reduce Inflammation

Cannabis is widely-valued as a treatment for inflammation. Credit goes to both THC and CBD in that regard, but cannabidiol has some special anti-inflammatory properties of its own.

Specifically, cannabidiol binds with the endocannabinoid system to produce a response that reduces nerve inflammation. This is another of its "neuroprotective" qualities and a major reason why CBD is such an effective treatment for neurological diseases.

CBD Can Treat Mood Disorders

Post Traumatic Stress Disorder (PTSD) affects nearly 8 percent of all American's during their lifetime. Women are twice as likely as men to suffer from it. Finding an affordable, safe, and reliable treatment for PTSD would profoundly impact the lives of millions of Americans every year.

To that end, a pathbreaking 2013 study found that cannabidiol improved people's abilities to forget their traumatic memories. These findings are incredibly important and could be relevant for figuring out how cannabidiol can treat other anxiety and stress disorders.

What Can CBD Do For Recreational Users?

The topic of treating stress and anxiety sets us up perfectly to pivot to the importance of cannabidiol for recreational marijuana users.

One of the most awesome things about CBD for the recreational crowd is its ability to act as a kind of counterweight to THC. The passive, sustaining Yin to the active, creative Yang of THC if you will.

CBD Can Produce A Smoother, More Balanced High

When recreational users report a negative experience with weed, the issue almost always has to do with feelings of paranoia and anxiety. No doubt, any serious recreational user has been there. Today's weed can be incredibly potentin terms of THC. And that's not even mentioning concentrates.

High doses of THC can and do trigger negative mood alterations. And some people are just more sensitive to THC than others. For both people who accidentally got "too high," and those hypersensitive to THC, cannabidiol can help pump the breaks by inhibiting some of the toxicity of THC.

This is a really unique and little-understood mechanism covered under the entourage effect. But if you take a close look at dispensary products, you'll see plenty of strains, edibles, and concentrates that include a healthy dose of CBD in addition to high quantities of THC.

The reason for this is that cannabidiol works like an antidote to THC. It counters some of the stronger, stress-inducing effects of THC, leading to a smoother, more balanced high.

Hence, 1:1 strains or other products with a balanced blend of THC and CBD are super-popular among recreational cannabis consumers.

The Most Popular CBD Products Available Today

CBD Oils

Today, the most popular way to purchase products and consume cannabidiol is as an oil. Remember, though, that CBD oil can come from hemp or from marijuana plants, and quality can vary dramatically.

Health and Beauty Products

Additionally, topical ointments, which allow CBD to be absorbed through the skin, are also tremendously popular. Moisturizers infused with CBD extracts are dominating the health and skin care markets for therapeutic cannabis. As are other CBD-infused products like shampoos, facial cleansers and even deodorant.

Vaporizers

Vaping CBD extracts in the form of wax concentrate is another popular mode of consuming cannabidiol.

Edibles

And finally, there's the old standbys: edibles and tinctures for making CBD-infused foods and beverages.

The Future Of Cannabidiol: The Future Of Healing?

That's the rundown of what cannabidiol is, what it can do for you and the most popular ways to get your hands on it. As you can see, the future holds in store some exciting things for CBD, thanks to its seemingly bottomless promise as an effective and safe medicine.

Capable of fighting back against the most serious diseases, while also gentle enough to be a part of a daily health regimen, cannabidiol is truly one of the most remarkable compounds in the natural world.

And for this reason, cannabidiol (CBD) is driving innovation in the cannabis industry. Who would have guessed that the part of the plant that doesn't get you high become such a major player in today's cannabis revolution?

CHAPTER TWO

How much CBD is in a gummy?

First, it's important that you understand product concentrations.

Concentrations vary from 1 mg CBD per gummy to 25 or 50 mg each. If a bag of gummies has 500mg of CBD in a 30 count bottle, you can get an estimate of the number of milligrams per gummy bear. In this case about 17 mg in each.

Other times you will see brands list the milligrams in a "serving." Often a serving correlates to one CBD gummy.

Take time to get your dose right

Dosing guidelines are limited. The best advice is to start low and work your way up to a dose that is right for you. One online resource suggests 1-6 mg of CBD per 10 lbs of body weight. So a 200-pound man might take 20 to 120 mg of CBD. This could be broken out through the course of a day.

Consider concentration when dosing for different conditions. Dosing for anxiety (regular, lower doses) may be very different from dosing for sleep (single, higher doses). That's not medical advice. It's what we hear from people who use CBD.

Dosing is the #1 question brands get. It's the question we get most often. This point can't be overstated: there is no clear or prescriptive answer.

How your body reacts to CBD is unique. How your body reacts to edibles is especially unique. Also, whether you want to "feel relaxed" or simply take a daily supplement is up to you. A capsule may give your body cannabinoids that steadily absorb into your body over time. A CBD vape you'll feel right away. Oils are closer to vapes in how quickly they work, but they take time to get into your system. Don't immediately take more. The impact of CBD may be cumulative.

How to find the best CBD gummies

Like most other CBD edibles, gummies are made by breaking down industrial hemp plants and extracting their valuable active compounds. Heat is an important factor in this process, but temperatures that are too hot can degrade the amount of CBD that actually makes it into a gummy. Temperatures should not exceed 200 °F during the creation of CBD-infused gummies, although it's very hard for consumers to find out how a particular product was specifically made. If you're serious about your CBD consumption, contact reputable brands or search their websites to see if they have information about how their CBD gummies are produced.

Other than purchasing from a company that properly heats their CBD, here's what else you can look for when choosing a CBD gummy that's right for you:

• Non-GMO products with organic sugars, flavors, and natural colors

• Third party testing, which provides an accurate description of ingredients

• Clearly stated CBD potency so you know how many milligrams are in each gummy

• Whether the CBD was extracted from hemp or marijuana (each one is a different strain of cannabis, but marijuana has more THC)

CBD Gummies—What's Real and What's Fake

There's a lot of misleading information on the internet that makes it even more confusing to find important details pertaining to CBD products. For example, several different websites claim that CBD gummies will take effect in a certain time frame. Some say it can take up to 2 hours, while others say you won't feel anything from CBD until 4 to 6 hours after consumption. Clearly, there are some discrepancies that need to be addressed.

The real answer is that everyone has a different metabolism, and there is no guarantee that CBD will have a certain effect on you. Generally, you can expect CBD gummies to work faster on an empty stomach than after eating a big meal, but it could take anywhere from half an hour to 3 hours (possibly more) for your endocannabinoid system to absorb all of the CBD.

Once you eat a CBD gummy, it may not always be apparent when it has started to work. CBD doesn't necessarily elicit a particular feeling, instead it reduces unwanted symptoms for a sense of overall well-being. The effects from a CBD gummy can last for hours, but exactly how long will depend on the potency of the product and how quickly your body absorbs the compound.

FAQs about CBD gummies

Is CBD safe?

According to the World Health Organization, CBD "is generally well tolerated, with a good safety profile." You should speak to your doctor about how CBD may interact with any medications you're currently taking.

Are CBD gummies legal in the United States?

In a word, yes, but there can be some confusion depending on where you live. For the majority of the country, it is legal to sell and purchase CBD as long as the THC percentage is less than .3%, and you're at the age of 18 or older.

Will I get high from eating CBD gummies?

No, CBD gummies are different than edibles made from marijuana and they will not get you high. There is little to no THC in these small treats. You may feel a sense of relaxation or notice that your symptoms have been alleviated, but you will not have any psychoactive effects like other THC-heavy edibles.

How many CBD gummies should I eat?

The answer to this question is going to be different for every person, and it will also depend on the type of gummies that you use. If you are new to CBD, start with gummies that have a smaller percentage of CBD, and only take one at a time. You won't feel the effects of CBD until your digestive system has started to break down the gummy. For this reason, it's important that you don't ingest too much CBD at once. It won't start to take effect until some time afterward, and after you eat a gummy there's really no way to undo the digestive process once it has started.

Will I fail a drug test if I eat CBD gummies?

Drug tests are looking for THC, and CBD contains no more than 0.3% of THC. This makes it highly unlikely that you would test positive for marijuana on a drug test. Most CBD is derived from hemp plants rather than marijuana plants, which further decreases the likelihood that THC would affect a drug test. However, if you consume a massive amount of CBD, there is a chance that trace amounts of THC are present in your urine. This could result in a false positive, even though no amount of CBD produces psychoactive effects like THC. According to the U.S. Drug Test Center, as long as you take less than 2,000 mg of CBD in a day you should be safe.

If you're still worried about a drug test and want to stay on the safe side, you can ensure that you'll pass with THC-free gummies and CBD isolates. These products only contain cannabidiol, rather than other terpenes and cannabinoids from the cannabis plant.

Where can I buy CBD gummies?

It's easy to find CBD hemp products all over the internet, just make sure that you are doing your research before purchasing anything that you intend to eat. Lab test results and accurate ingredient lists are a good place to start. This way you'll know exactly how much CBD is going into your body, along with anything else that was used to make the gummies.

The Differences Between CBD Gummies and CBD Oil

In the large world of Kratom consumers, there are a select few who cross the bridge and enjoy CBD gummies along with their Kratom.

However, there are other people in the Kratom community who have never tried CBD gummies, but are very curious to learn what CBD gummies have to offer. We want to discuss how it can benefit you to include a gummy regiment into your daily routine. Being a consistent Kratom consumer, you probably already understand the importance of plant-based practices in your daily wellness routines.

CBD Gummies Are The Same As CBD Oil!

One of the many questions we get about our CBD products is, "what's the difference between your gummies and your CBD oil?"

It's a fair enough question and we want to make sure you understand the differences between the two so you can make an educated selection today.

First of all, CBD stands for "Cannabidiol", and is one of the most comprehensive compounds in the cannabis plant. Let's get one thing clear, there are hundreds of different cannabinoids, but not all cannabinoids are equal to each other. Customers have responded that our CBD products are very satisfying, bringing calmness, clarity, and great relief to their day.

But, let's get back on track, we are here to discuss the one known as cannabidiol (CBD). The more research scientists perform on cannabidiol, the more evidence they find that could revolutionize the medical industry.

The hemp plant is where both CBD oil and our gummies are harvested from. Hemp is in the Cannabis plant family, and you already know the popular plant harvested from cannabis – marijuana.

However, while cannabidiol can come from both the hemp and marijuana plant, the hemp plant is known for producing CBD because hemp produces high quantities of CBD and low quantities of THC. On the other hand, the marijuana plant is known for its high quantity of THC and low quantity of CBD. So essentially, in origin, gummies and CBD oil come from the same plant, which is hemp.

Both gummies and oil activate the endocannabinoid system in your body. The chemical marriage that happens during this process is beneficial and valuable to your anatomy. The endocannabinoid system is an almost magical process which runs deep throughout the human body and touches a lot of our main response systems. Scientists are still discovering even more positive reactions when the body interacts with CBD, and what a healthy endocannabinoid system means to you.

CBD Gummies Are Different From CBD Oil

When comparing CBD oil to CBD gummies, there is a difference. I have personally received many emails (this past week) where our community is wondering which of these would be better trying first.

There are many scientific reasons behind why you should buy CBD oil and/or CBD gummies, but you are probably wondering which one would benefit you the most? It's important to know the differences between the two.

Here are the differences:

Our gummies are made from the isolation of the CBD compound. CBD oil is made from every bit of the hemp plant. Let me explain.

When I say CBD gummies are made from isolate, this means it is pure CBD. We use a special process of extraction to isolate the compound so you are getting CBD and CBD only.

On the other hand, our CBD oil is made from the entire hemp plant. This means a certain amount of THC does come with the oil when it's harvested. In case you're wondering, our CBD oil contains the legal limit of THC (.03%).

Increasing Popularity of CBD Gummies

The CBD product market is exploding across the world. There are numerous new products that are coming to market almost every day in this largely unregulated industry. Unfortunately, this means that there's no shortage of businesses that are trying to cash in on the "CBD craze." This has resulted in ineffective, low-quality CBD gummies that are being sold at inflated prices by fly-by-night companies.

Green Roads CBD gummies are one of the few genuinely trusted sources of CBD products available on the market at the moment. All of the Green Roads raw compounds are third-party lab tested for quality, and the fact that the company tests for potency and purity – and posts the results online – just goes to show that they are night and day ahead of the competition. Green Roads also uses Colorado-certified organic hemp, and is the only company we know of that employs a full-time licensed pharmacist to oversee all product manufacturing.

Another way that Green Roads stands out from its competitors is its return policy: You may return your products for a full refund if you aren't satisfied within 30 days. Many other CBD companies won't allow you to return opened products, or they will offer a partial refund for a shorter period of time.

One of the reasons that Green Roads has been so successful is because of this unrivaled, extraordinarily high level of customer service.

Another brand we've personally had success with is Hemp Bombs CBD gummies. Hemp Bombs pride themselves on sourcing and importing only the highest grade organically-certified European hemp. And not only do they adhere to the strict European hemp practices, but they have also set up their own quality control standards, which includes third-party lab testing.

Side Effects of CBD Gummies

While CBD gummies side effects have not been studied in a clinical or laboratory setting, there is some research that has been done on the side effects of CBD in general. According to Very Well

Health, CBD may result in things like mood and appetite changes, diarrhea, dizziness, and drowsiness. On a potentially more serious level, some have suggested that CBD oil may affect liver enzyme levels.

While the consumption of CBD gummies seems to have few notable side effects (according to our research of anecdotal evidence), it would still be wise to practice caution as some candies offer potent cannabinoid doses. For example, even though CBD gummies come in small sizes, they can contain as much as 25 mg or more of active compounds – definitely enough to make one drowsy or potentially dizzy.

Also, keep in mind that many of the best CBD gummies are made with corn syrup and processed sugars, so it's important to read the label of any product before consumption – especially if you're a diabetic and/or are particularly concerned with the "nutritional value" of what you're eating.

How to pick the right CBD gummies

Edibles are a mainstay of the cannabis community. They are a discrete and tasty option that many people love. CBD edibles come in many forms, too. There are gummy bears, chocolates, caramels, and hard candies, to name a few. The great thing about CBD gummies, specifically, is that you can achieve a relaxing feeling without the psychoactive effects of a gummy that contains THC.

But the tricky thing about gummies is knowing how much to take. We have said that CBD works differently for everyone, and this is especially true for edibles.

When it comes to edibles, your metabolism is another variable in the equation. CBD gummies take effect when they are digested, and everyone metabolizes food at different rates.

If you digest slowly, a gummy may take a while to work but the relief can linger for a long time. For others, an edible may hit them quickly and dissipate soon. Everyone is different.

Be smart:

Most people are taking CBD to achieve some therapeutic value. People want to empower their endocannabinoid system and achieve more physiological balance. Don't you think the restorative power of CBD is offset if you eat a handful of sugar? Think about how much CBD is in a gummy. If you need to eat a handful of candy to get a proper dose of CBD then you haven't taken a supplement—you've had a snack

The best way to vet a CBD brand is to:

- Look for test results: All brands should post recent, detailed test results on their website. Because testing is unregulated and irregular, Remedy Review does its own testing. If we have recently tested a product and it passed, you'll see the Remedy Review Seal.

- Call the brands: A brand should stand by its product. Some brands offer full refunds if you're not satisfied. If it's hard to get ahold of a real person at a cannabis brand, move on to another. There's plenty of caring people out there who want to help you get better.

- Do some math: Look closely at price and CBD content on edibles. If you're buying gummy bears that have 1mg of CBD each you might need to eat 20 to feel any relaxation. If you're taking CBD to sleep, you don't want to eat a bag of gummy bears before bed.

To help us compile this buyer's guide we spoke with

- Product managers

- Consumer advocates

- Patients and consumers

The common theme of all our conversations is that buyers need to be careful. You should do your research and try multiple brands. CBD as a market is growing much faster than regulations or oversight. It's up to consumers to protect themselves.

Note

You should consult a professional when making decisions about your health, especially if you have a pre-existing medical condition. You should also know that despite strong anecdotal evidence to support the impact of CBD, clinical trials are limited and these products have not been evaluated by the FDA. We aim to be a measured voice, to help you get good info. But our advice is editorial—not medical. Talk to your doctor.

Our Review Methodology

People are taking CBD gummies for sleep, pain, and anxiety. They are looking for relief. We believe products with this kind of health potential should be safe and of great quality. We also believe the brands that make edibles should be transparent.

We also understand comparing brands is difficult. That's why we want to point out 6 Core Principles that you can use to easily review CBD oil brands. Use these key differentiators to make simple, personal decisions about what CBD brand is right for you.

These are the 6 things we believe customers should use to compare CBD brands and find the best CBD gummies.

But this information only provides a foundation. We've added an additional layer of scrutiny to the buying process.

Once you narrow your list of brands, consider some other things.

Is the CBD gummy full-spectrum or an isolate?

We believe full-spectrum products have greater therapeutic value. Some people talk about the "entourage effect," or multiple cannabinoids working together. Experts we talk to support the idea of whole-plant therapy. Look for brands that believe in full-spectrum or broad-spectrum CBD.

Does this brand operate in a state where marijuana is legal?

States that have legalized marijuana have more standardized regulations. The industry in these places has infrastructure and processes in place. States that only allow limited cultivation of industrial hemp simply have less resources to scrutinize product development.

Do I want a brand that does one thing great or has everything I need?

Consider product diversity. Some people like to shop brands who have a very narrow expertise. Other people like access to a wide variety of CBD products all in one place. The main thing to look out for is white labeling.

Is the company who sells everything accountable for the manufacturing of those products or are they a storefront?

Does this brand have assistance programs and military discounts available?
Medicine and supplements are expensive. We like seeing brands who make access to their products easier.

CHAPTER THREE

CBD Gummies for Anxiety

CBD Anxiety & Depression Studies

Recent data revealed that 1 in 5 Americans took some type of psychiatric medication recently, meaning anxiety and depression are much more common than we'd like to talk about. Most of what we know about CBD and mental health comes from animal studies and small-scale human experiments. However, a growing body of evidence along with thousands of anecdotal reports suggests CBD can improve symptoms of anxiety and mood disorders.

Today, CBD is used to relieve symptoms of numerous conditions, from anxiety and mental illness to chronic pain. Chronic stress is often a primary trigger of anxiety, and animal studies show us that CBD can calm the stress-response and nervous system. Further experimentson mice and humans show us that CBD also has properties that can relax the muscles and blood vessels, even during stress. It also exhibits a natural calming effect on the mind, which could aid the onset of sleep and reduce symptoms of anxiety or depression.

Researchers believe this effect occurs when CBD binds with the 5-HT1A neuro-receptor. This receptor is essentially like a signaling hub in the brain for emotions and is also the main target of most modern antidepressants.

One of the most notable studies on CBD's effects on anxiety disorders in humans comes from a trial on the fear of public speaking. Compared to a placebo, CBD reduced the physical markers of stress-related anxiety and participants reported fewer symptoms of the phobia.

Several peer-reviewed analysis also now confirm and validate the study's results indicating CBD as a potential drug for anxiety disorders.

Using CBD Gummies For Anxiety & Depression

Taking CBD for sleep, anxiety, and depression can be as simple as snacking on a few tasty Gummies once or twice per day. CBD-infused Gummies are made using all-natural ingredients and non-GMO, organic CBD hemp concentrate produced by super-critical CO_2 extraction. Similar to taking chewable vitamins, Gummies offer a safe, effective way to easily take cannabidiol as a daily supplement. You can find them available in a range of potencies from 5mg-25mg and are typically sold in 30-60 count bottles.

CBD gummies come in a variety of dosages, typically offering between 5mg and 25mg per candy. CBD is non-toxic and non-intoxicating, which means that you can't overdose from eating too many gummies. Unlike with THC edibles, you don't have to worry about experiencing anxiety or paranoia from eating too many CBD Gummies.

There is no exact dosage of CBD for any particular condition or ailment, but it's generally recommended to begin taking CBD gummies in smaller, low dosages. You can increase the dosage as needed once you've observed how CBD may affect your symptoms. Similar to eating grapefruit, CBD could alter the way your body metabolizes certain types of medications. Always consult with your doctor first for treating serious health conditions.

Why Do People Choose CBD Gummies Over Other Forms Of CBD?

When it comes to cannabidiol, if all things are held constant (like product quality) the major differences in products boils down to administration/consumption methods. For example, tinctures are dropped under the tongue and the CBD is absorbed sublingually. Gummies however, are eaten and the CBD is absorbed through the digestion process.

The most popular reason for using gummies over tinctures or other forms of CBD is by far, the taste. Many people find the earthy flavors of oils to be unappealing. CBD gummies however, taste great. People also find that using the gummies is a little more discreet than other forms, and they can administer their CBD in public more freely.

When comparing the effects of tinctures over edibles, consumers typically notice a faster and stronger effect when using tinctures. For anxiety or depression issues, they can be great in high-stress moments where the onset of panic begins, using CBD oil sublingually might help elevate issues in moments, rather than waiting for the CBD to be digested.

Some anecdotal reports suggest CBD gummies offer longer lasting but milder effects than some other forms of CBD. However, consumers do report that using CBD gummies and edibles for anxiety is extremely effective as well. This is because edibles tend to have a "milder" effect, but last longer as the CBD goes through the digestion process to be absorbed into the bloodstream. People with anxiety issues tend to notice that they handle the rigors and stresses of daily life much better throughout the day when using edibles over tinctures.

Best CBD Gummies You Should Buy To Beat Anxiety

Where the market is saturated with brands selling CBD and its products, we have done your homework for you and have curated a list of 5 best online brands who you should buy CBD gummies from.

1) RedStarCBD

RedStarCBD manufactures CBD gummies which are 100% natural, free from toxins and THC-free. Brig THC free these gummies do not get you high. You can enjoy the therapeutic effects of CBD and have gummy bears' fun experience as well. High-quality, full-spectrum CBD is infused in these gummies to ensure the delivery of CBD at the cellular level.

Following a range of gummies is available at RedStarCBD. Each pack contains 5 pieces with 20mg of CBD in each. Hence, each pack contains 100 mg of CBD.

- Apple gummy rings infused with CBD

- Peach gummy rings infused with CBD

- Watermelon gummy rings infused with CBD

- Blue Raz Gummy RingsSour Neon Gummy bears

- Sour Neon Gummy Worms infused with CBD

- Black and Red Raspberries infused with CBD

- Strawberry Gummies infused with CBD

- Cherry Cola gummies infused with CBD

- Watermelon gummies infused with CBD

- Arctic muscle roll on infused with CBD

- Sour 40's gummies infused with 40mg of CBD infused with CBD

40's gummies have 5 pieces in each pack. Each gummy has 40 mg CBD which makes a total of 200 mg CBD in each pack.

Many people are having complaints of insomnia, back pain and anxiety, bought these gummies and felt a visible change after the initial use.

2) CBDFx

CBD gummies made by CBDFxare 100% vegan and potent. Following CBD gummy products are available at the online shop:

i- CBD gummy bears 300mg

This is the most natural CBD gummy bear available in the market. It is free from GMO, corn syrup or any artificial sweeteners. The product is made from

CBD extracted from organically grown hemp plant having full spectrum CBD oil.

Moreover, the berry flavour adds to the fun that you have while eating these gummies. Each container contains 60 gummy bears with5 mg CBD in each gummy. Pure CBD oil is infused in the gummies.

ii- CBD gummies 8ct pouch

This is also 100% natural and conations no GMO or corn syrup. It is 100% vegan and contains no artificial flavours or sweeteners. Each container has 60 gummy bears with 5mg CBD oil in each. Pure CBD oil used!

3) Green Roads CBD gummy bears:

Green Roads provide CBD gummy bears which are natural and have assorted flavours. Each bag contains 30 gummy bears with 10 mg CBD in each.

The gummy bears manufactured by Green Roads are a combination of a number of ingredients including corn syrup, gelatin, sugar, citric acid, FD&C, flavours, anhydrous hemp oil extract, pharmaceutical grade CBD, Broad spectrum CBD 6% and candy gummies.

4) Hemp Bombs

Hemp bomb is also a runner-up in the list of top CBD gummies selling the online brand. It has the following product to offer:

CBD gummies by Hemp Bomb delivers the strong health benefits as promised. These naturally manufactured gummies provide you with an effortless way to introduce this additional and essential health supplement in your daily routine diet and health regime.

The CBD infused in these gummies is certified pure cannabidiol and is extracted from hemp plant with an eco-forward methodology and minimum human footprint.CBD in these gummies has numerous therapeutic benefits and lack the psychoactive effects of THC which makes CBD a very useful supplement.

The gummies also contain additional ingredients including L-Theanine, Passiflora, Scutellaria, Sugar, Gelatin, Corn syrup, Citric Acid, Silicon Dioxide, Calcium Lactate, and Natural& Artificial Flavors.

Each container by Hemp Bomb contains 5 CBD gummies with 15 mg CBD in each. The product is laboratory tested and contains no THC. There is no risk of failed drug test with these CBD gummies.

5) Pure Kana

Last but not the least! Pure Kana brings you one of the most potent forms of CBD infused gummies. These are 100% vegan and contain no GMO. There is no THC, no getting high and no failed drug tests.

The gummies are specially designed to help you relax and set your mind free of all anxieties and stresses.

High-quality natural ingredients have been used in the manufacture of these gummies including organic evaporated cane juice, organic white grape juice concentrate, organic corn syrup, pectin sodium citrate, ascorbic acid, citric acid, natural flavours and colours.

Each bottle of Pure Kana CBD gummies contains 20 gummies with 25 mg CBD in each. This makes a total of 200mg CBD in each bottle.

CHAPTER FOUR

CONCLUSION

For those of dealing with anxiety and depression, CBD edibles may hold the key to less worrying, better sleep, and an overall improved quality of life. But out of all the products that exist on the market, CBD gummies are probably the most popular edibles.

The CBD oil used to produce these edibles is extracted from carefully-selected types of cannabis, with low THC and a high concentration of cannabidiol. CBD-based products are part of a different category of medicinal marijuana, one that does not place emphasis on the psychoactive effects of the plant, but rather the curative properties of marijuana. Those who use these natural products as an alternative to medication or other treatments that may involve unpleasant side effects claim amazing results. From chronic pain and inflammation to sleep disorders, anxiety, and depression, CBD gummies seem to be the new "miracle cure."

But there's absolutely nothing mystical or magical about this chemical compound. In fact, people have been using it for thousands of years as a remedy for various conditions. Recently, scientists have begun to explore the physical and psychological effects CBD, with promising results.

Who knows? Maybe CBD gummies and other edibles may become the next breakthrough in mental health.

CBD market is drowning in the list of online brands selling CBD gummies. However, the top 5 brands selling quality gummies are listed above. Moreover, although CBD has a number of therapeutic effects, an excess of everything is bad! It is always recommended that you should consult your medical practitioner first in order to make sure if when and how you should take these supplements. Moreover, keep these away from the reach of children!